Table of Contents

Introduction

Cancer is one of the leading causes of death worldwide. But studies suggest that simple lifestyle changes, such as following a healthy diet, could prevent 30–50% of all cancers. Growing evidence points to certain dietary habits increasing or decreasing cancer risk. What's more, nutrition is thought to play an important role in treating and coping with cancer. This book covers everything you need to know about the link between diet and cancer.

Cancer

Cancer causes cells to divide uncontrollably. This can result in tumors, damage to the immune system, and other impairment that can be fatal. In the United States, an estimated 15.5 million people with a history of cancer were living as of January 1, 2016, according to a 2018 report from the American Cancer Society. Cancer is a broad term. It describes the disease that results when cellular changes cause the uncontrolled growth and division of cells. Some types of cancer cause rapid cell growth, while others cause cells to grow and divide at a slower rate. Certain forms of cancer result in visible growths called tumors, while others, such as leukemia, do not. Most of the body's cells have specific functions and fixed lifespans. While it may sound like a bad thing, cell death is part of a natural and beneficial phenomenon called apoptosis. A cell receives instructions to die so that the body can replace it with a newer cell that functions better. Cancerous cells lack the components that instruct them to stop dividing and to die. As a result, they build up in the body, using oxygen and nutrients that would usually nourish other cells. Cancerous cells can form tumors, impair the immune system and cause other changes that prevent the body from functioning regularly. Cancerous cells may appear in one area, then spread via the lymph nodes. These are clusters of immune cells located throughout the body.

Types Of Cancer

The most common type of cancer in the U.S. is breast cancer, followed by lung and prostate cancers, according to the National Cancer Institute, which excluded nonmelanoma skin cancers from these findings. Each year, more than 40,000 people in the country receive a diagnosis of one of the following types of cancer:

• bladder

- colon and rectal

- endometrial

- kidney

- leukemia

- liver

- melanoma

- non-Hodgkin's lymphoma

- pancreatic

- thyroid

Other forms are less common. According to the National Cancer Institute, there are over 100 types of cancer.

Cancer development and cell division

Doctors classify cancer by:

- its location in the body

- the tissues that it forms in

For example, sarcomas develop in bones or soft tissues, while carcinomas form in cells that cover internal or external surfaces in the body. Basal cell carcinomas develop in the skin, while adenocarcinomas can form in the breast. When cancerous cells spread to other parts of the body, the medical term for this is metastasis. A person can also have more than one type of cancer at a time.

Risk Factors And Causes Of Cancer

Anything that may cause a normal body cell to develop abnormally potentially can cause cancer. Many things can cause cell abnormalities and have been linked to cancer development. Some cancer causes remain unknown while other cancers have environmental or lifestyle triggers or may develop from more than one known cause. Some may be developmentally influenced by a person's genetic makeup. Many patients develop cancer due to a combination of these factors. Although it is often difficult or impossible to determine the initiating event(s) that cause a cancer to develop in a specific person, research has provided clinicians with a number of likely causes that alone or in concert with other causes, are the likely candidates for initiating cancer. The following is a listing of major causes and is not all-inclusive as specific causes are routinely added as research advances:

• Chemical or toxic compound exposures: Benzene, asbestos, nickel, cadmium, vinyl chloride, benzidine, N-nitrosamines, tobacco or cigarette smoke (contains at least 66 known potential carcinogenic chemicals and toxins), asbestos, and aflatoxin

• Ionizing radiation: Uranium, radon, ultraviolet rays from sunlight, radiation from alpha, beta, gamma, and X-ray-emitting sources

• Pathogens: Human papillomavirus (HPV), EBV or Epstein-Barr virus, hepatitis viruses B and C, Kaposi's sarcoma-associated herpes virus (KSHV), Merkel cell polyomavirus, Schistosoma spp., and Helicobacter pylori; other bacteria are being researched as possible agents.

• Genetics: A number of specific cancers have been linked to human genes and are as follows: breast, ovarian, colorectal, prostate, skin and melanoma; the specific genes and other details are beyond the scope of this general article so the reader is referred to the National Cancer Institute for more details about genetics and cancer.

It is important to point out that most everyone has risk factors for cancer and is exposed to cancer-causing substances (for example, sunlight, secondary cigarette smoke, and X-rays) during their lifetime, but many individuals do not develop cancer. In addition, many people have the genes that are linked to cancer but do not develop it. Why? Although researchers may not be able give a satisfactory answer for every individual, it is clear that the higher the amount or level of cancer-causing materials a person is exposed to, the higher the chance the person will develop cancer. In addition, the people with genetic links to cancer may not develop it for similar reasons (lack of enough stimulus to make the genes function). In addition, some people may have a heightened immune response that controls or eliminates cells that are or potentially may become cancer cells. There is evidence that even certain dietary lifestyles may play a significant role in conjunction with the immune system to allow or prevent cancer cell survival. For these reasons, it is difficult to assign a specific cause of cancer to many individuals.

Recently, other risk factors have been added to the list of items that may increase cancer risk. Specifically, red meat (such as beef, lamb, and pork) was classified by the International Agency for Research on Cancer as a high-risk agent for potentially causing cancers; in addition, processed meats (salted, smoked, preserved, and/or cured meats) were placed on the carcinogenic list. Individuals that eat a lot of barbecued meat may also increase risk due to compounds formed at high temperatures. Other less defined situations that may increase the risk of certain cancers include obesity, lack of exercise, chronic inflammation, and hormones, especially those hormones used for replacement therapy. Other items such as cell phones have been heavily studied. In 2011, the World Health Organization classified cell phone low energy radiation as "possibly carcinogenic," but this is a very low risk level that puts cell phones at the same risk as caffeine and pickled vegetables.

Proving that a substance does not cause or is not related to increased cancer risk is difficult. For example, antiperspirants are considered to possibly be related to breast cancer by some investigators and not by others. The official stance by the NCI is "additional research is needed to investigate this relationship and other factors that may be involved." This unsatisfying conclusion is presented because the data collected so far is contradictory. Other claims that are similar require intense and expensive research that may never be done. Reasonable advice might be to avoid large amounts of any compounds even remotely linked to cancer, although it may be difficult to do in complex, technologically advanced modern societies.

Cancer Symptoms And Sign

Cancer often has no specific symptoms, so it is important that people limit their risk factors and undergo appropriate cancer screening. Most cancer screening is specific to certain age groups and your primary care doctor will know what screening to perform depending on your age. People with risk factors for cancer (for example, smokers, heavy alcohol use, high sun exposure, genetics) should be acutely aware of potential cancer symptoms and be evaluated by a physician if any develop. The best way to fight cancers is by prevention (eliminating or decreasing risk factors) and early detection. Cancer treatment advances every year and combined with early detection has made many cancers treatable. Consequently, individuals need to know which symptoms might point to cancer. People should not ignore a warning symptom that might lead to early diagnosis and possibly to a cure. Cancer gives most people no symptoms or signs that exclusively indicate the disease.

Unfortunately, every complaint or symptom of cancer can be explained by a harmless condition as well. Some cancers occur more frequently in certain age groups. If certain symptoms occur or persist, however, a doctor should be seen for further evaluation. Some common symptoms that may occur with cancer are as follows:

• Persistent cough or blood-tinged saliva: These symptoms usually represent simple infections such as bronchitis or sinusitis. They could be symptoms of lung cancer or head and neck cancer. Anyone with a nagging cough that lasts more than a month or with blood in the mucus that is coughed up should see a doctor.

• A change in bowel habits: Most changes in bowel habits are related to your diet and fluid intake. Doctors sometimes see pencil-thin stools with colon cancer. Occasionally, cancer exhibits continuous diarrhea. Some people with cancer feel as if they need to have a bowel movement and still feel that way after they have had a bowel movement. If any of these abnormal bowel complaints last more than a few days, they require evaluation. Any significant change in bowel habits that cannot be easily explained by dietary changes could be cancer-related and needs to be evaluated.

• Blood in the stool: A doctor always should investigate blood in your stool. Hemorrhoids frequently cause rectal bleeding, but because hemorrhoids are so common, they may exist with cancer. Therefore, even when you have hemorrhoids, you should have a doctor examine your entire intestinal tract when you have blood in your bowel movements. With some individuals, X-ray studies may be enough to clarify a diagnosis. Colonoscopy is usually recommended. Routine colonoscopy, even without symptoms, is recommended once you are 50 years old. Sometimes when the source of bleeding is entirely clear (for example, recurrent ulcers), these studies may not be needed.

• Unexplained anemia (low blood count): Anemia is a condition in which people have fewer than the expected number of red blood cells in their blood. Anemia should always be investigated. There are many kinds of anemia, but blood loss almost always causes iron deficiency anemia. Unless there is an obvious source of ongoing blood loss, this anemia needs to be explained. Many cancers can cause anemia, but bowel cancers most commonly cause iron deficiency anemia. Evaluation should include endoscopy or X-ray studies of your upper and lower intestinal tracts.

• Breast lump or breast discharge: Most breast lumps are noncancerous tumors such as fibroadenomas or cysts. But all breast lumps need to be thoroughly investigated for the possibility of breast cancer. A negative mammogram result is not usually sufficient to evaluate a breast lump. Your doctor needs to determine the appropriate X-ray study which might include an MRI or an ultrasound of the breast. Generally, diagnosis requires a needle aspiration or biopsy (a small tissue sample). Discharge from a breast is common, but some forms of discharge may be signs of cancer. If discharge is bloody or from only one nipple, further evaluation is recommended. Women are advised to conduct monthly breast self-examinations.

• Lumps in the testicles: Most men (90%) with cancer of the testicle have a painless or uncomfortable lump on a testicle. Some men have an enlarged testicle. Other conditions, such as infections and swollen veins, can also cause changes in your testicles, but any lump should be evaluated. Men are advised to conduct monthly testicular self-examinations.

• A change in urination: Urinary symptoms can include frequent urination, small amounts of urine, and slow urine flow or a general change in bladder function. These symptoms can be caused by urinary infections (usually in women) or, in men, by an enlarged prostate gland. Most men will suffer from harmless prostate enlargement as they age and will often have these urinary symptoms. These symptoms may also signal prostate cancer. Men experiencing urinary symptoms need further investigation, possibly including blood tests and a digital rectal exam. The PSA blood test, its indications, and interpretation of results should be discussed with your health care provider. If cancer is suspected, a biopsy of the prostate may be needed. Cancer of the bladder and pelvic tumors can also cause irritation of the bladder and urinary frequency.

Diagnosing Cancer

Often, a diagnosis begins when a person visits a doctor about an unusual symptom. The doctor will talk with the person about his or her medical history and symptoms. Then the doctor will do various tests to find out the cause of these symptoms. But many people with cancer have no symptoms. For these people, cancer is diagnosed during a medical test for another issue or condition. Sometimes a doctor finds cancer after a screening test in an otherwise healthy person. Examples of screening tests include colonoscopy, mammography, and a Pap test. A person may need more tests to confirm or disprove the result of the screening test. For most cancers, a biopsy is the only way to make a definite diagnosis. A biopsy is the removal of a small amount of tissue for further study. Learn more about making a diagnosis after a biopsy.

Treatments Of Cancer

Innovative research has fueled the development of new medications and treatment technologies. Doctors usually prescribe treatments based on the type of cancer, its stage at diagnosis, and the person's overall health. Below are examples of approaches to cancer treatment:

• Chemotherapy aims to kill cancerous cells with medications that target rapidly dividing cells. The drugs can also help shrink tumors, but the side effects can be severe.

• Hormone therapy involves taking medications that change how certain hormones work or interfere with the body's ability to produce them. When hormones play a significant role, as with prostate and breast cancers, this is a common approach.

• Immunotherapy uses medications and other treatments to boost the immune system and encourage it to fight cancerous cells. Two examples of these treatments are checkpoint inhibitors and adoptive cell transfer.

• Precision medicine, or personalized medicine, is a newer, developing approach. It involves using genetic testing to determine the best treatments for a person's particular presentation of cancer. Researchers have yet to show that it can effectively treat all types of cancer, however.

• Radiation therapy uses high-dose radiation to kill cancerous cells. Also, a doctor may recommend using radiation to shrink a tumor before surgery or reduce tumor-related symptoms.

• Stem cell transplant can be especially beneficial for people with blood-related cancers, such as leukemia or lymphoma. It involves removing cells, such as red or white blood cells, that chemotherapy or radiation has destroyed.

Lab technicians then strengthen the cells and put them back into the body.

• Surgery is often a part of a treatment plan when a person has a cancerous tumor. Also, a surgeon may remove lymph nodes to reduce or prevent the disease's spread.

• Targeted therapies perform functions within cancerous cells to prevent them from multiplying. They can also boost the immune system. Two examples of these therapies are small-molecule drugs and monoclonal antibodies.

Doctors will often employ more than one type of treatment to maximize effectiveness.

Tips For Cancer Prevention

While your diet is central to preventing cancer, other healthy habits can further lower your risk:

• Be as lean as possible without becoming underweight. Weight gain, overweight and obesity increases the risk of a number of cancers, including bowel, breast, prostate, pancreatic, endometrial, kidney, gallbladder, esophageal, and ovarian cancers.

• Be physically active for at least 30 minutes every day. Physical activity decreases the risk of colon, endometrial, and postmenopausal breast cancer. Three 10-minute sessions work just as well, but the key is to find an activity you enjoy and make it a part of your daily life.

• Limit alcoholic drinks. Limit consumption to no more than two drinks a day for men and one a day for women.

• Where possible, aim to meet nutritional needs through diet alone, instead of trying to use supplements to protect against cancer.

• It is best for mothers to breastfeed exclusively for up to 6 months and then add other liquids and foods. Babies who are breastfed are less likely to be overweight as children or adults.

After treatment, cancer survivors should follow the recommendations for cancer prevention. Follow the recommendations for diet, healthy weight, and physical activity from your doctor or trained professional.

Cancer And Diet

The development of cancer, in particular, has been shown to be heavily influenced by your diet. Many foods contain beneficial compounds that could help decrease the growth of cancer.

Broccoli

Broccoli contains sulforaphane, a plant compound found in cruciferous vegetables that may have potent anticancer properties. One test-tube study showed that sulforaphane reduced the size and number of breast cancer cells by up to 75%. Similarly, an animal study found that treating mice with sulforaphane helped kill off prostate cancer cells and reduced tumor volume by more than 50%. Some studies have also found that a higher intake of cruciferous vegetables like broccoli may be linked to a lower risk of colorectal cancer. One analysis of 35 studies showed that eating more cruciferous vegetables was associated with a lower risk of colorectal and colon cancer. Including broccoli with a few meals per week may come with some cancer-fighting benefits. However, keep in mind that the available research hasn't looked directly at how broccoli may affect cancer in humans. Instead, it has been limited to test-tube, animal and observational studies that either investigated the effects of cruciferous vegetables, or the effects of a specific compound in broccoli.Thus, more studies are needed.

Carrots

Several studies have found that eating more carrots is linked to a decreased risk of certain types of cancer.For example, an analysis looked at the results of five studies and concluded that eating carrots may reduce the risk of stomach cancer by up to 26%. Another study found that a higher intake of carrots was associated with 18% lower odds of developing prostate cancer.One study analyzed the diets of 1,266 participants with and without lung cancer. It found that current smokers who did not eat carrots were three times as likely to develop lung cancer, compared to those who ate carrots more than once per week. Try incorporating carrots into your diet as a healthy snack or delicious side dish just a few times per week to increase your intake and potentially reduce your risk of cancer. Still, remember that these studies show an association between carrot consumption and cancer, but don't account for other factors that may play a role.

Beans

Beans are high in fiber, which some studies have found may help protect against colorectal cancer. One study followed 1,905 people with a history of colorectal tumors, and found that those who consumed more cooked, dried beans tended to have a decreased risk of tumor recurrence. An animal study also found that feeding rats black beans or navy beans and then inducing colon cancer blocked the development of cancer cells by up to 75%. According to these results, eating a few servings of beans each week may increase your fiber intake and help lower the risk of developing cancer.However, the current research is limited to animal studies and studies that show association but not causation. More studies are needed to examine this in humans, specifically.

Berries

Berries are high in anthocyanins, plant pigments that have antioxidant properties and may be associated with a reduced risk of cancer. In one human study, 25 people with colorectal cancer were treated with bilberry extract for seven days, which was found to reduce the growth of cancer cells by 7%. Another small study gave freeze-dried black raspberries to patients with oral cancer and showed that it decreased levels of certain markers associated with cancer progression. One animal study found that giving rats freeze-dried black raspberries reduced esophageal tumor incidence by up to 54% and decreased the number of tumors by up to 62%. Similarly, another animal study showed that giving rats a berry extract was found to inhibit several biomarkers of cancer. Based on these findings, including a serving or two of berries in your diet each day may help inhibit the development of cancer. Keep in mind that these are animal and observational studies looking at the effects of a concentrated dose of berry extract, and more human research is needed.

Cinnamon

Cinnamon is well-known for its health benefits, including its ability to reduce blood sugar and ease inflammation. In addition, some test-tube and animal studies have found that cinnamon may help block the spread of cancer cells. A test-tube study found that cinnamon extract was able to decrease the spread of cancer cells and induce their death. Another test-tube study showed that cinnamon essential oil suppressed the growth of head and neck cancer cells, and also significantly reduced tumor size. An animal study also showed that cinnamon extract induced cell death in tumor cells, and also decreased how much tumors grew and spread. Including 1/2–1 teaspoon (2–4 grams) of cinnamon in your diet per day may be beneficial in cancer prevention, and may come with other benefits as well, such as reduced blood sugar and decreased inflammation.However, more studies are needed to understand how cinnamon may affect cancer development in humans.

Nuts

Research has found that eating nuts may be linked to a lower risk of certain types of cancer. For instance, a study looked at the diets of 19,386 people and found that eating a greater amount of nuts was associated with a decreased risk of dying from cancer. Another study followed 30,708 participants for up to 30 years and found that eating nuts regularly was associated with a decreased risk of colorectal, pancreatic and endometrial cancers. Other studies have found that specific types of nuts may be linked to a lower cancer risk. For example, Brazil nuts are high in selenium, which may help protect against lung cancer in those with a low selenium status. Similarly, one animal study showed that feeding mice walnuts decreased the growth rate of breast cancer cells by 80% and reduced the number of tumors by 60%. These results suggest that adding a serving of nuts to your diet each day may reduce your risk of developing cancer in the future. Still, more studies in humans are needed to determine whether nuts are responsible for this association, or whether other factors are involved.

Olive Oil

Olive oil is loaded with health benefits, so it's no wonder it's one of the staples of the Mediterranean diet. Several studies have even found that a higher intake of olive oil may help protect against cancer. One massive review made up of 19 studies showed that people who consumed the greatest amount of olive oil had a lower risk of developing breast cancer and cancer of the digestive system than those with the lowest intake. Another study looked at the cancer rates in 28 countries around the world and found that areas with a higher intake of olive oil had decreased rates of colorectal cancer. Swapping out other oils in your diet for olive oil is a simple way to take advantage of its health benefits. You can drizzle it over salads and cooked vegetables, or try using it in your marinades for meat, fish or poultry. Though these studies show that there may be an association between olive oil intake and cancer, there are likely other factors involved as well. More studies are needed to look at the direct effects of olive oil on cancer in people.

Turmeric

Turmeric is a spice well-known for its health-promoting properties. Curcumin, its active ingredient, is a chemical with anti-inflammatory, antioxidant and even anticancer effects. One study looked at the effects of curcumin on 44 patients with lesions in the colon that could have become cancerous. After 30 days, 4 grams of curcumin daily reduced the number of lesions present by 40%. In a test-tube study, curcumin was also found to decrease the spread of colon cancer cells by targeting a specific enzyme related to cancer growth. Another test-tube study showed that curcumin helped kill off head and neck cancer cells. Curcumin has also been shown to be effective in slowing the growth of lung, breast and prostate cancer cells in other test-tube studies. For the best results, aim for at least 1/2–3 teaspoons (1–3 grams) of ground turmeric per day. Use it as a ground spice to add flavor to foods, and pair it with black pepper to help boost its absorption.

Citrus Fruits

Eating citrus fruits such as lemons, limes, grapefruits and oranges has been associated with a lower risk of cancer in some studies. One large study found that participants who ate a higher amount of citrus fruits had a lower risk of developing cancers of the digestive and upper respiratory tracts. A review looking at nine studies also found that a greater intake of citrus fruits was linked to a reduced risk of pancreatic cancer. Finally, a review of 14 studies showed that a high intake, or at least three servings per week, of citrus fruit reduced the risk of stomach cancer by 28%. These studies suggest that including a few servings of citrus fruits in your diet each week may lower your risk of developing certain types of cancer. Keep in mind that these studies don't account for other factors that may be involved. More studies are needed on how citrus fruits specifically affect cancer development.

Flaxseed

High in fiber as well as heart-healthy fats, flaxseed can be a healthy addition to your diet. Some research has shown that it may even help decrease cancer growth and help kill off cancer cells. In one study, 32 women with breast cancer received either a flaxseed muffin daily or a placebo for over a month. At the end of the study, the flaxseed group had decreased levels of specific markers that measure tumor growth, as well as an increase in cancer cell death. In another study, 161 men with prostate cancer were treated with flaxseed, which was found to reduce the growth and spread of cancer cells. Flaxseed is high in fiber, which other studies have found to be protective against colorectal cancer. Try adding one tablespoon (10 grams) of ground flaxseed into your diet each day by mixing it into smoothies, sprinkling it over cereal and yogurt, or adding it to your favorite baked goods.

Tomatoes

Lycopene is a compound found in tomatoes that is responsible for its vibrant red color as well as its anticancer properties. Several studies have found that an increased intake of lycopene and tomatoes could lead to a reduced risk of prostate cancer. A review of 17 studies also found that a higher intake of raw tomatoes, cooked tomatoes and lycopene were all associated with a reduced risk of prostate cancer. Another study of 47,365 people found that a greater intake of tomato sauce, in particular, was linked to a lower risk of developing prostate cancer. To help increase your intake, include a serving or two of tomatoes in your diet each day by adding them to sandwiches, salads, sauces or pasta dishes. Still, remember that these studies show there may be an association between eating tomatoes and a reduced risk of prostate cancer, but they don't account for other factors that could be involved.

Garlic

The active component in garlic is allicin, a compound that has been shown to kill off cancer cells in multiple test-tube studies. Several studies have found an association between garlic intake and a lower risk of certain types of cancer. One study of 543,220 participants found that those who ate lots of Allium vegetables, such as garlic, onions, leeks and shallots, had a lower risk of stomach cancer than those who rarely consumed them. A study of 471 men showed that a higher intake of garlic was associated with a reduced risk of prostate cancer. Another study found that participants who ate lots of garlic, as well as fruit, deep yellow vegetables, dark green vegetables and onions, were less likely to develop colorectal tumors. However, this study did not isolate the effects of garlic. Based on these findings, including 2–5 grams (approximately one clove) of fresh garlic into your diet per day can help you take advantage of its health-promoting properties. However, despite the promising results showing an association between garlic and a reduced risk of cancer, more studies are needed to examine whether other factors play a role.

Fatty Fish

Some research suggests that including a few servings of fish in your diet each week may reduce your risk of cancer. One large study showed that a higher intake of fish was associated with a lower risk of digestive tract cancer. Another study that followed 478,040 adults found that eating more fish decreased the risk of developing colorectal cancer, while red and processed meats actually increased the risk. In particular, fatty fish like salmon, mackerel and anchovies contain important nutrients such as vitamin D and omega-3 fatty acids that have been linked to a lower risk of cancer. For example, having adequate levels of vitamin D is believed to protect against and reduce the risk of cancer. In addition, omega-3 fatty acids are thought to block the development of the disease. Aim for two servings of fatty fish per week to get a hearty dose of omega-3 fatty acids and vitamin D, and to maximize the potential health benefits of these nutrients. Still, more research is needed to determine how fatty fish consumption may directly influence the risk of cancer in humans.

Foods That Increase The Risk Of Cancer

It's difficult to prove that certain foods cause cancer. However, observational studies have repeatedly indicated that high consumption of certain foods may increase the likelihood of developing cancer.

Sugar and Refined Carbs

Processed foods that are high in sugar and low in fiber and nutrients have been linked to a higher cancer risk. In particular, researchers have found that a diet that causes blood glucose levels to spike is associated with an increased risk of several cancers, including stomach, breast and colorectal cancers. One study in over 47,000 adults found that those who consumed a diet high in refined carbs were almost twice as likely to die from colon cancer than those who ate a diet low in refined carbs. It's thought that higher levels of blood glucose and insulin are cancer risk factors. Insulin has been shown to stimulate cell division, supporting the growth and spread of cancer cells and making them more difficult to eliminate. In addition, higher levels of insulin and blood glucose can contribute to inflammation in your body. In the long term, this can lead to the growth of abnormal cells and possibly contribute to cancer. This may be why people with diabetes — a condition characterized by high blood glucose and insulin levels — have an increased risk of certain types of cancer. For example, your risk of colorectal cancer is 22% higher if you have diabetes. To protect against cancer, limit or avoid foods that boost insulin levels, such as foods high in sugar and refined carbs.

Processed Meat

The International Agency for Research on Cancer (IARC) deems processed meat a carcinogen — something that causes cancer. Processed meat refers to meat that has been treated to preserve flavor by undergoing salting, curing or smoking. It includes hot dogs, ham, bacon, chorizo, salami and some deli meats. Observational studies have found an association between consuming processed meat and an increased cancer risk, particularly colorectal cancer. A large review of studies found that people who ate large amounts of processed meat had a 20–50% increased risk of colorectal cancer, compared to those who ate very little or none of this type of food. Another review of over 800 studies found that consuming just 50 grams of processed meat each day — around four slices of bacon or one hot dog — raised the risk of colorectal cancer by 18%. Some observational studies have also linked red meat consumption to an increased cancer risk. However, these studies often don't distinguish between processed meat and unprocessed red meat, which skews results. Several reviews that combined results from multiple studies found that the evidence linking unprocessed red meat to cancer is weak and inconsistent.

Overcooked Food

Cooking certain foods at high temperatures, such as grilling, frying, sautéing, broiling and barbequing, can produce harmful compounds like heterocyclic amines (HA) and advanced glycation end-products (AGEs). Excess buildup of these harmful compounds can contribute to inflammation and may play a role in the development of cancer and other diseases. Certain foods, such as animal foods high in fat and protein, as well as highly processed foods, are most likely to produce these harmful compounds when subjected to high temperatures. These include meat — particularly red meat — certain cheeses, fried eggs, butter, margarine, cream cheese, mayonnaise, oils and nuts. To minimize cancer risk, avoid burning food and choose gentler cooking methods, especially when cooking meat, such as steaming, stewing or boiling. Marinating food can also help.

Dairy

Several observational studies have indicated that high dairy consumption may increase the risk of prostate cancer. One study followed almost 4,000 men with prostate cancer. Results showed that high intakes of whole milk increased the risk of disease progression and death. More research is needed to determine possible cause and effect. Theories suggest that these findings are due to an increased intake of calcium, insulin-like growth factor 1 (IGF-1) or estrogen hormones from pregnant cows — all of which have been weakly linked to prostate cancer.

Plant-Based Diets May Help Protect Against Cancer

Higher intake of plant-based foods has been associated with a reduced risk of cancer. Studies have found that people who follow a vegetarian or vegan diet have a reduced risk of developing or dying from cancer. In fact, a large review of 96 studies found that vegetarians and vegans may have an 8% and 15% lower risk of cancer, respectively. However, these results are based on observational studies, making it difficult to identify possible reasons. It's likely that vegans and vegetarians eat more vegetables, fruits, soy and whole grains, which may protect against cancer. Moreover, they're less likely to consume foods that have been processed or overcooked — two factors that have been linked to a higher cancer risk.

Keto Diet And Cancer

Keto Diet May Help Fight Certain Cancer Tumors

• Maintaining blood sugar levels can be helpful for your overall health.

• Early research also points to the benefits of keeping blood sugar levels low to help fight cancer.

• Past research has found that certain tumors may rely on high glucose levels.

Keeping blood sugar levels even throughout the day may help you avoid afternoon energy crashes. It might also ward off or help you manage diabetes. Now, early research published in the journal Cell Reports suggests that restricting your blood sugar might also help combat certain cancerous tumor growths. Researchers from the University of Texas at Dallas restricted blood sugar levels in mice by feeding them a ketogenic diet — one that's high in fat, moderate in protein, and low in carbs — and by giving them a diabetes drug that prevents the kidneys from reabsorbing glucose in the blood. The combination of the diet and diabetes drug didn't shrink the lung and esophageal cancers in the mice, but it did keep them from progressing. "Both the ketogenic diet and the pharmacological restriction of blood glucose by themselves inhibited the further growth of squamous cell carcinoma tumors in mice with lung cancer," Jung-Whan "Jay" Kim, PhD, corresponding author of the study and an assistant professor of biological sciences at UT Dallas, said in a press release. Both elements actually showed promise independent of one another, too. "The key finding of our new study in mice is that a ketogenic diet alone does have some tumor-growth inhibitory effect in squamous cell cancer," Kim said.

"When we combined this with the diabetes drug and chemotherapy, it was even more effective." However, Kim and his colleagues report that the keto diet and drug combination had no effect on non-squamous cell cancers. The research is in the extremely early stages. It's unclear if these results could be replicated in humans. But it joins a growing body of evidence finding that certain diets, including the keto diet, may act as a complementary therapy for some people undergoing cancer treatment.

A Secondary Finding Targets Sugar

This finding in particular suggests certain tumors might be susceptible to glucose restriction. It helps confirm earlier research by Kim and colleagues. Their 2017 study indicated that a certain type of cancer called squamous cell carcinoma (SCC) was particularly reliant on glucose to sustain itself and survive. As part of their research, Kim and investigators also took blood samples from 192 people who had SCC of the lung or esophagus, plus blood samples from 120 people with lung adenocarcinoma, another type of cancer. They measured the blood glucose levels in the samples and divided them by whether they were above or below 120 mg/dL, a common clinical measure of diabetes in blood sugar. "Surprisingly, we found a robust correlation between higher blood-glucose concentration and worse survival among patients with squamous cell carcinoma," Kim said. "We found no such correlation among the lung adenocarcinoma patients. This is an important observation that further implicates the potential efficacy of glucose restriction in attenuating squamous-cell cancer growth," he said. In other words, people who had SCC and a high blood glucose level had worse survival rates compared to people who had other types of cancer. This secondary finding indicates that blood glucose levels may also have an impact on the progression of cancer. Managing blood glucose levels during treatment may be an effective way to enhance conventional methods of cancer treatment. "Manipulating host glucose levels would be a new strategy that is different from just trying to kill cancer cells directly," Kim said. "I believe this is part of a paradigm shift from targeting cancer cells themselves. Immunotherapy is a good example of this, where the human immune system is activated to go after cancer cells."

The Keto Diet's Potential As Cancer Treatment

Cancer treatment and care have seen a shift in recent years. While conventional treatments like surgery, chemotherapy, and radiation are still the primary means for eliminating cancerous tumors, researchers are seeking out complementary methods that may help stop the growth of cells, or even help defeat them. These methods aren't thought of as a way to replace traditional therapies like radiation. Instead, they'd be an additional aid in the fight against cancer. In fact, one 2014 study already identified the keto diet "as an adjuvant therapy to conventional radiation and chemotherapies." In addition to helping regulate blood sugar levels, a keto diet could selectively induce metabolic oxidative stress in cancer cells. This could help make the cells more sensitive to treatments like chemotherapy and radiation. "Ketogenic diets are known to interfere with tumor growth in more ways than one," said

Dr. William Li, author of "Eat to Beat Disease: The New Science of How Your Body Can Heal Itself." "Reducing glucose takes away a fuel source for cancer cells. Unlike healthy cells, abnormal cancer cells have difficulty adapting metabolically to a low glucose situation, compromising their ability to survive." Li further explained, "But a ketogenic diet also triggers a chain reaction of at least three other cancer-fighting mechanisms. Less glucose means cells produce less IGF-1, a protein growth signal for cancer. Ketogenic diets also lower the tumor's ability to produce another growth signal called VEGF.

Tumors use this signal to grow a private blood supply. By cutting off the tumor blood supply, an effect called anti-angiogenesis, cancer cells become starved and can't grow." But the ketogenic diet shouldn't be considered standard care, says Quintin Pan, PhD, deputy scientific director at University Hospitals Seidman Cancer Center. It's too early to know if the benefits outweigh possible risks. "The anticancer benefits of a keto diet for cancer patients remain an open question and need to be addressed in a controlled clinical trial," Pan told Healthline. Pan also points out that the keto diet specifically is notoriously difficult to maintain. People undergoing cancer treatment should always talk with their doctor before trying a new strict diet and discuss potential issues that may arise for them. Many people receiving chemotherapy are nauseous; they may not be able to stick with a very strict diet. "Strict adherence to a keto diet is challenging, especially for cancer patients. And also, keto diets may lead to potential health risks," Pan said. "It is important for cancer patients to have a conversation with their clinician team, doctor, and dietitian before starting on a keto diet." While there still needs to be more research, some experts are advising certain patients to see if the keto diet is right for them. Elena Villanueva, DC, a functional holistic medicine expert and founder of Modern Holistic Health, says some treatment facilities are beginning to use the diet because of anecdotal reports and preliminary data that show promising signs. "For those battling with cancer and for those who are in remission, the adaptation of a healthy ketogenic diet is showing many benefits," she said. "Several oncology centers around the country have implemented ketogenic diets combined with standard cancer treatments because of the anticancer effects from eliminating sugars from the diet."

Recipes

Sheet Pan Eggs With Veggies And Parmesan

• Servings: 6

• Prep Time: 5 minutes

• Cook Time: 15 minutes

Ingredients:

• 12 large eggs, whisked

• Salt and pepper

• 1 small red pepper, diced

• 1 small yellow onion, chopped

• 1 cup diced mushrooms

• 1 cup diced zucchini

• 1 cup freshly grated parmesan cheese

Instructions:

• Preheat the oven to 350°F and grease a rimmed baking sheet with cooking spray.

• Whisk the eggs in a bowl with salt and pepper until frothy.

• Stir in the peppers, onions, mushrooms, and zucchini until well combined.

• Pour the mixture in the baking sheet and spread into an even layer.

• Sprinkle with parmesan and bake for 12 to 15 minutes until the egg is set.

• Let cool slightly, then cut into squares to serve.

Nutrition Info: 215 calories, 14g fat, 18.5g protein, 5g carbs, 1g fiber, 4g net carbs

Bacon Cheeseburger Soup

• Servings: 4

• Prep Time: 10 minutes

• Cook Time: 15 minutes

Ingredients:

- 4 slices uncooked bacon

- 8 ounces ground beef (80% lean)

- 1 medium yellow onion, chopped

- 1 clove garlic, minced

- 3 cups beef broth

- 2 tablespoons tomato paste

- 2 teaspoons Dijon mustard

- Salt and pepper

- 1 cup shredded lettuce

- ½ cup shredded cheddar cheese

Instructions:

- Cook the bacon in a saucepan until crisp then drain on paper towels and chop.

- Reheat the bacon fat in the saucepan and add the beef.

- Cook until the beef is browned, then drain away half the fat.

• Reheat the saucepan and add the onion and garlic – cook for 6 minutes.

• Stir in the broth, tomato paste, and mustard then season with salt and pepper.

• Add the beef and simmer on medium-low for 15 minutes, covered.

• Spoon into bowls and top with shredded lettuce, cheddar cheese and bacon.

Nutrition Info: 315 calories, 20g fat, 27g protein, 6g carbs, 1g fiber, 5g net carbs

Grilled Pesto Salmon With Asparagus

• Servings: 4

• Prep Time: 5 minutes

• Cook Time: 15 minutes

Ingredients:

• 4 (6-ounce) boneless salmon fillets

• Salt and pepper

• 1 bunch asparagus, ends trimmed

• 2 tablespoons olive oil

• ¼ cup basil pesto

Instructions:

• Preheat a grill to high heat and oil the grates.

• Season the salmon with salt and pepper, then spray with cooking spray.

• Grill the salmon for 4 to 5 minutes on each side until cooked through.

• Toss the asparagus with oil and grill until tender, about 10 minutes.

• Spoon the pesto over the salmon and serve with the asparagus.

Nutrition Info: 300 calories, 17.5g fat, 34.5g protein, 2.5g carbs, 1.5g fiber, 1g net carbs